100 Plus Homemade Essential Oil Beauty Recipes

Aromatherapy Preparations For Skin, Lip And Hair Care (Body Scrubs, Perfumes, Lotions, Creams, Deodorants, Bath Salts, Soaps And More)

Sandy Comfort

ISBN-13: 978-1499506303

DEDICATION

This book is dedicated to all my sisters across the globe. You are more beautiful than you think!

TABLE OF CONTENTS

Read Other Books By Sandy Comfort

100 Plus Simple Homemade Organic Body Scrub Recipes: For Face And Body Exfoliating (Available on Amazon)

INTRODUCTION

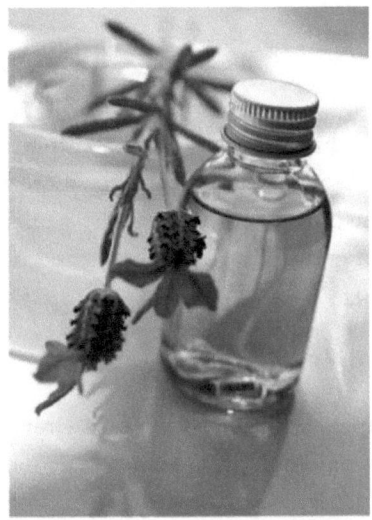

Nowadays, people are more health conscious than before. This is evident in the clamor for everything organic and natural. Whether it is our foods, clothing or beauty products, a large number of us now stay away from artificial additives having embraced the growing trend to go natural.

Using essential oil in our homemade beauty products such as perfumes, lotions, creams, cleansers, body scrubs and deodorants is one of the best ways to get the best out of our products. Extracted from plants, bark, roots, wood, flowers or seeds, essential oils are natural, highly concentrated oils with powerful antioxidant properties.

On my own part, I started experimenting with essential oils after being dissatisfied with the smells of store-bought products. In addition to the smells, these products contain chemicals that cause considerable damage to our skin. They are also very expensive. Then again, essential oils do a lot more than make you smell nice. They offer tremendous healing and purifying benefits.

Essential oils penetrate the skin easily. Within a few minutes, they are carried all through the blood and tissues. They increase the amount of oxygen that goes to the pineal and the pituitary glands. This ultimately increases the release of endorphins, antibodies and neurotransmitters which are healthy for the body.

Essential oil has multiple medicinal properties. Unlike most of our drugs that are meant for just one remedy, lavender essential oil for example, has analgesic, anti-inflammatory, sedative and antispasmodic properties. This means that it is suitable for pain, stress, sleeping and muscle cramps.

If kept in a cool dark place, essential oils usually last for up to 2 years. Only a few drops are required so they are very affordable.

Other benefits of essential oil:

- Prevent hair loss, improves hair quality

- Regenerate skin

- Support the immune system

- Sooth and promote healing of wounds, sunburn and scrapes

- Sooth digestive upsets

- Sooth emotional issues

- Promote healthy thyroid and hormone function

Essential oil tips to remember:

- Do not use internally.

- Do not apply directly on your skin but dilute with carrier oil.

- Keep out children's reach.

- Avoid contact with eyes.

- Use only pure essential oils; stay away from synthetic fragrances.

- To avoid degradation and rancidity, store essential oils properly.

- Before experimenting with any oil, try to know its properties, precautions and dose.

- Do not use on children, pregnant women and the elderly

Use only essential oils that are safe for your skin.

1. HOMEMADE INVIGORATING BATH RECIPES

There is simply no reason to have a plain and unexciting bath time experience when there are several invigorating bath recipes to choose from. Containing essential oils, salts and other natural ingredients, these recipes are a healthy addition to your body. The inclusion of essential oils into your bath helps to hydrate and soften your skin as well as improve its tone and texture.

Bath salts contain anti-inflammatory properties and when combined with essential oils, you will have the opportunity of doubling the relief, rejuvenation and bliss that you'll enjoy. There are other bath recipes listed below such as bath bombs, bath cookies and bath teas. Take your pick and enjoy a healthy bath.

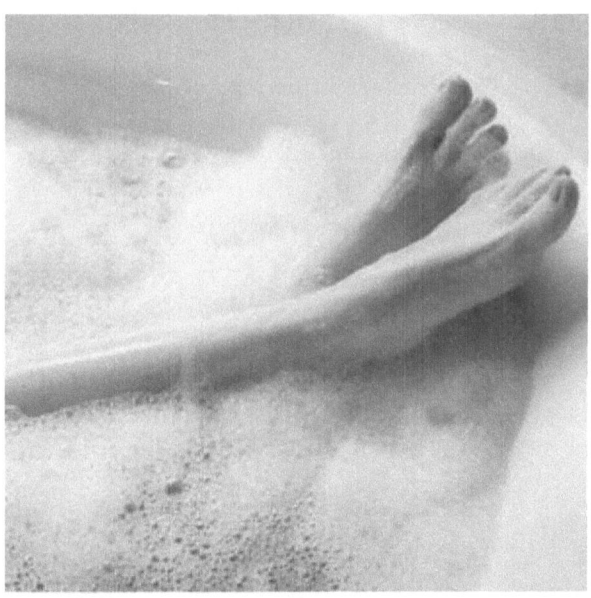

BATH OILS

Simple Aromatherapy Bath Oil

Ingredients:

Essential oil of choice (15-30 drops)

Olive oil (1 1/2 oz)

Canola oil (1 oz)

Sesame oil (1 oz)

Almond oil (3 oz)

Wheat germ oil (1/2 oz)

Directions:

1.   Fill a small- mouth jar with all the carrier oils.

2.   Leave 1 /8 inch of space at the top.

3.   Gradually add the essential oil.

4.   use a tight lid to cap the jar and shake thoroughly

5.   Use 2 teaspoons of oil per bath.

Blissful Oil Bath

Ingredients:

Sandalwood (10 drops)

Jasmine (5 drops)

Rose (5 drops)

Bergamot (5 drops)

Any of these base oils: Jojoba, Castor, Almond or simple Sunflower (4tbs)

Directions:

1.   Pour base oil into a glass jar or bottle

2.   Add essential oil. Cover and shake thoroughly.

3.   Store in a dark place and leave for 2weeks to mature.

4.   Once matured, add 1 tablespoon of the scented oil to the bath.

5.   Swish to disburse.

6.   Enjoy your blissful oil bath and remain happy.

Sensuous Oil Bath

Ingredients:

Jasmine (20 drops)

Orange (8 drops)

Any of these base oils: Jojoba, Castor, Almond or simple Sunflower (4tbs)

Directions:

1.   Pour base oil into a glass jar or bottle.

2.   Add essential oil. Cover and shake thoroughly.

3.   Store in a dark place and leave for 2weeks to mature.

4.   Once matured, add 1 tablespoon of the scented oil to the bath.

5.   Swish to disburse.

6.   Enjoy your sensual oil bath.

Revitalizing Oil Bath

Ingredients:

Geranium (12 drops)

Sandalwood (6 drops)

Lemon (6 drops)

Clary Sage (2 drops)

Any of these base oils: Jojoba, Castor, Almond or simple Sunflower (4tbs)

Directions

1.   Pour base oil into a glass jar or bottle

2.   Add essential oil. Cover and shake thoroughly.

3.   Store in a dark place and leave for 2weeks to mature.

4.   Once matured, add 1 tablespoon of the scented oil to the bath

5.   Swish to disburse

6.   Enjoy your revitalizing oil bath to relive stress and depression.

Relaxing Oil

Ingredients:

Sandalwood (12 drops)

Orange (8 drops)

Rose (4 drops)

Pine (2 drops)

Lemon (2 drops)

Any of these base oils: Jojoba, Castor, Almond or simple Sunflower (4tbs)

Directions

1.   Pour base oil into a glass jar or bottle

2.   Add essential oil. Cover and shake thoroughly.

3.   Store in a dark place and leave for 2weeks to mature.

4.   Once matured, add 1 tablespoon of the scented oil to the bath

5.   Swish to disburse

6.   Enjoy your relaxing oil bath to relive stress and depression

Shampoo Bath Oil

Ingredients:

Essential oil of choice (10 drops)

Mild baby shampoo (4 tbsp)

Almond or Sunflower Oil (125ml)

 Note:

Baby shampoo is an effective carrier that helps to quickly and evenly disburse your oils.

Direction:

1.   Pour base oil into a glass jar.

2.   Add the shampoo and shake well

3.   Add essential oil, shake well

4.   Leave for 2 weeks to mature but keep way from daylight.

5.   Once matured, add 2 tablespoons per bath and swish to disperse

6.   Enjoy your bath.

Alcohol Bath Oil

Ingredients:

Castor Oil (100ml)

Vodka or brandy (4 tbsp)

 Essential oils of choice (10 drops)

Note:

Spirits help in the quick and even distribution of the oil.

Direction

1.   Pour the castor oil into a glass jar.

2.   Add the spirit and shake well

3.   Add essential oil, shake well

4.   Leave for 2 weeks to mature but keep way from daylight.

5.   Once matured, add 2 tablespoons per bath and swish to disperse

6.   Enjoy your bath.

Here are my 10 best singular bath oil recipes:

Treatment	Essential oil	Quantity
Depression	Bergamot oil	5 drops
Stress or fatigue	Jasmine	8 drops
Soothing and relaxing	Lavender	10 drops
Insomnia or itchy skin	Chamomile	7 drops
Sensual and mellowing a great aphrodisiac	Sandalwood	8 drops
Happiness and romantic pleasure	Rose	10 drops
Relaxing, uplifting and energizing	Geranium	10 drops
hypnotic with antidepressant properties	Neroli	7 drops
energizing and invigorating	Patchouli	5 drops
sedative and mood sweetening	Frankincense	8 drops

BATH SALTS

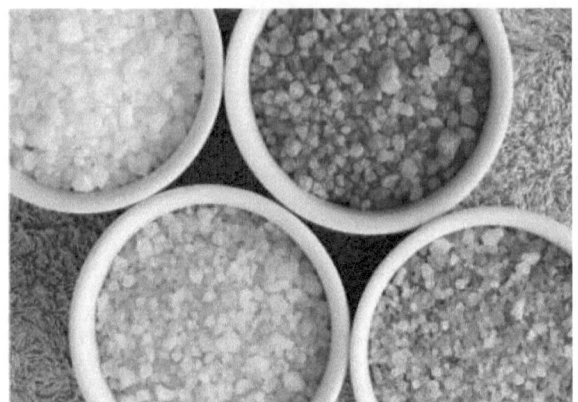

Lemon Bath Salt Recipe

Ingredients:

Fine grain Sea Salt (1 cup)

Epsom Salt (1 cup)

Dendritic salt (ideal for making scented bath salts, 3 tbsp)

Lemon essential oil (1/2 tsp)

Vanilla Extract (1/2 tsp)

Yellow 5 liquid dye (5 drops)

Directions:

1.   Pour the fine grain Sea Salt and the Epsom Salt into a large stainless steel mixing bowl and then set aside.

2.	In a separate but smaller mixing bowl, pour in the dendritic salt and add the vanilla extract and the lemon essential oil.

3.	Mix very thoroughly and then add this mixture to the salts in the large stainless steel mixing bowl.

4.	Mix thoroughly. Add yellow dye to the salt mixture and continue to mix well until the color is even throughout

5.	Either use immediately or package well.

Margarita Bath Salt Recipe

Ingredients:

Epsom salts (1 cup)

Green food coloring (4-5 drops)

Lime essential oil (10 drops)

Directions:

1.	Combine all the ingredients: Epsom salts, essential oil and coloring and mix well.

2.	Pour into in a small glass jar and seal.

3.	 Leave it to set for several days.

4.	Store in plastic bags or decorative jars.

5.	Add bath salts into hot running or warm bath water.

6.	Soak liberally.

Seaside Bath Salt Soak

Ingredients:

Epsom Salt (210 grams)

Kelp Powder (9 grams)

Powdered Grapefruit Peel (6 grams)

Spirulina Powder (3 grams)

Olive Oil (40 grams)

Rosemary Essential Oil (60 drops)

Juniper Essential Oil (30 drops)

Eucalyptus Essential Oil (20 drops)

Notes:

1.   Grapefruit Peel powder, Kelp powder and Spirulina powder improves skin tone and promotes the synthesis of new collagen.

2.   Epsom salt is ideal for soothing, relaxing and relieving sore muscles.

3.   You may also use Sea Salt just add a few scoops of it to warm running bath water.

4.   Be careful because this product contains oil and oil is slippery.

Directions:

1.   Mix all the ingredients in a small bowl.

2.   Transfer to a glass jar and use within 60 days.

3.   This recipe may cause the bath surface to become very slippery so be careful while using it.

Aromatherapy Bath Salts Recipe

Ingredients:

Epsom salts (2 1/2 cups)

Baking Soda (1 cup)

Citric Acid (1/2 cup)

Sweet Almond Oil (2 1/2 tsp)

Ginger, peppermint and eucalyptus essential Oils (about 60 drops)

Directions

1.   In a mixing bowl, combine all the dry ingredients until the entire clumps are broken.

2.   Mix your essential oils and set aside. Add the sweet almond oil to your essential oils recipe.

3.   Mix them all together and blend thoroughly.

4.   Package in a plastic bag.

Oatmeal, Milk And Honey Salt Bath

Ingredients:

Powdered full cream/whole milk (4 cups)

Ground oats (1 cup)

Ground plain, raw almonds (1 cup)

Baking soda (1/2 cup)

Sea salt (1 cup)

Honey (2 cups)

Vanilla Essential oil (4 drops)

Notes:

Milk : Contains lactic acid which helps in breaking down and dissolving the proteins that hold together the dead skin cells. These dead skin cells must be removed in order for fresh new ones to resurface leading to a total youthful looking skin.

Honey : can absorb and retain moisture and this is why it is an essential ingredient in this recipe. It has natural antibacterial antifungal and antioxidant properties as well and this facilitates healing of different skin problems.

Oatmeal as well as baking soda is a wonderful exfoliant helps to soothe and heal rashes, sunburn and skin irritations. Grind oatmeal so that it will easily blend with the bath water and milk. It also draws toxin.

Directions:

1.   Combine the sea salt, almond, oats, bathing soda and milk and then mix thoroughly.

2.   Dissolve 4 cups of this powdered mixture in warm bath water (alternatively, you may pour the mix mixture into a cheesecloth bag, a clean sock or coffee filter, tie it securely with a string and then soak in the bath water).

3.   Add the honey and vanilla essential oil in the bath water and mix it thoroughly so it completely dissolves.

4.   Soak your body in the bath for about 15 minutes.

5.   Rinse out the milk body under a warm shower.

6.   Gently dry your skin with a clean towel.

Ocean Bath Salts

Ingredients:

Epsom salt (1 cup)

Glycerin (2 tbsp)

Baking soda (1 cup)

Vanilla (4 drops)

Blue food coloring (4 drops)

Essential oil (3 drops)

Directions:

1.   Combine dry ingredients and mix well.

2.   Add scents and color one at a time.

3.   Continue to stir until thoroughly mixed.

4.   Break up any clumps.

5.   Keep on mixing until a semi fine powder is formed.

6.   Add glycerin and mix well.

OTHER BATH RECIPES

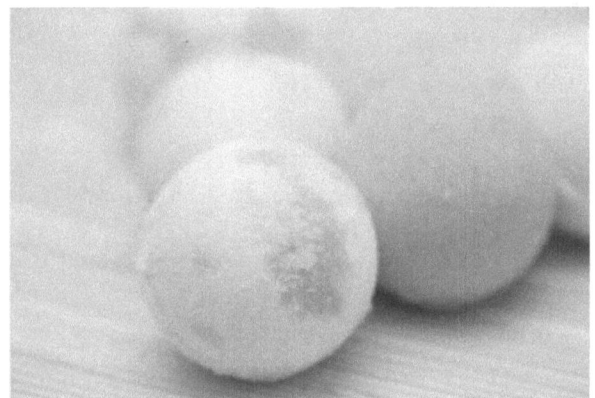

Plain Milk Bath

Ingredients:

Non-fat powdered milk (2 cups)

Cornstarch (1 cup)

Essential oil (5 drops)

Directions:

1.   Mix ingredients well.

2.   Add 1/2 cup to hot bath and enjoy a refreshing bath.

Lavender Milk Bath

Ingredients:

Powdered milk (1 cup)

Lavender essential oil (2-3 drops)

Directions:

1.   Mix ingredients together

2.   Add to bath.

Meadow Milk Bath

Ingredients:

Finely sifted Powdered Milk (4 oz)

Citric Acid (2 oz)

Corn starch (2 oz)

Grapefruit Seed Oil (30 drops)

Jasmine essential oil (60 drops)

Directions

1.   Blend the corn starch and powdered milk and then sift.

2.   Mix the grapefruit seed oil and Jasmine in Citric Acid.

3.   Make sure the oils are well blended in the Citric Acid.

4.   Add the Citric Acid blend to the milk/corn starch blend.

5.   Use 3 tablespoons to each bath.

Relaxing Bath Tea

Ingredients:

Lavender flowers (4 oz.)

Chamomile flowers (4 oz.)

Calendula petals (2 oz)

Bulgarian Lavender EO (20 drops)

Directions

1.   Combine ingredients and package.

Silky Body Wash

Ingredients:

Shea butter (1 tbsp)

Aloe Vera gel (1/4 cup)

Guar gum (3/4 tsp)

Castile Soap (3/4 cup)

Essential oils of choice (25 drops)

Directions:

1.   Melt the Shea butter over low heat.

2.   Add aloe Vera gel to the Shea butter and warm together.

3.   Add gum and use a whisk to stir thoroughly.

4.   Add the soap base.

5.   Mix thoroughly in a blender to get the gum fully distributed.

6.   After blending, your wash will appear foamy but will settle in a couple of hours.

7.   Pour some in your bath or use in the shower.

Lavender & Chamomile Bath Melts

Ingredients:

Organic Shea butter (50g)

Organic cocoa butter (50g)

Lavender essential oil (2 drops)

Dried lavender flowers (1 tsp)

Organic chamomile tea (1 tsp)

Directions:

1.   Thinly grate the cocoa butter and pour in a glass bowl. Add the Shea butter as well.

2.   Place your glass bowl on a pan of hot water, stir until it melts then remove from heat.

3.   Sprinkle organic chamomile tea into the mix. Add the dried lavender and stir thoroughly.

4.   Pour the molten mix carefully into silicone moulds (ice cube trays can also be used).

5.   Add the lavender essential oil to the moulds.

6.   Refrigerate your melts for an hour so its hardens

7.   Pop the melts from their mould and store in a fine glass jar.

How To Use:

1.   Pop a bath melt in a warm bath and then wait till it dissolves.

2.   The cocoa butter may make your bath a little slippery so you've got to be careful

3.   However, you can put your bath melt in a muslin cloth bag if you do not want the chamomile and lavender flowers to cover your bath.

Scented Bath Bombs

Ingredients:

Baking soda (1 1/2 cups)

Citric acid 1/2 cup

Essential oil of choice (8 drops)

Sweet almond oil (1/2 tsp)

Food coloring of choice (2 drops)

Directions

1.   Combine all the ingredients.

2.   Press into mould or muffin tin of choice.

3.   Release from mould.

4.   Wrap in plastic wraps and tie with a ribbon.

2. HOMEMADE SOAP RECIPES

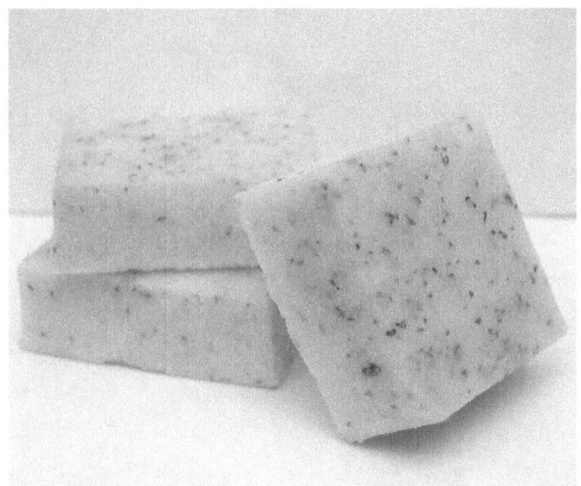

Homemade Lemon Soap

Ingredients:

Goat's milk soap base (13 cubes)

Lemon essential oil

Lemon zest of 3-4 lemons (optional)

Directions:

1.   Cut the soap into cubes.

2. Melt soap for about 2 minutes using a large pyrex measuring cup.

3. As soon as soap cubes turn liquid, add the lemon zest and some drops of the lemon essential oil and stir well.

4. Pour into soap molds. Leave for one hour to harden.

5. Press mold to release soap.

Seaweed Soap

Ingredients:

Clear soap base (32 ounces)

Dried seaweed (6-8 pieces)

Extra virgin olive oil (1 teaspoon)

Lemon essential oil (1.5 teaspoons)

Lavender essential oil (1 teaspoon)

Dash of green mica

Mold: 3 part Ziploc, divided rectangle mold

Directions:

1. Place seaweed pieces into mold.

2. Slice the soap base into tiny cubes.

3. Add the essential oils, colorant and olive oil just before the soap is completely melted, stir well.

4. Slowly pour into the molds.

5. Leave soap in freezer or fridge to harden. It may remain in at room temperature, however.

6. Remove from molds.

7. Once the soap is at room temperature, cut and wrap.

Hand Wash Liquid Soap

Ingredients:

Liquid Soap (1 cup)

Water (1 cup)

Essential oils of choice (8 drops)

Directions:

1. mix ingredients together

2. pour into a bottle

3. shake thoroughly

Antibacterial & Antiviral Hand Wash Soap

Ingredients:

Liquid Soap (1 cup)

Water (1 cup)

Essential oils of choice (8 drops)

Tea Tree oil (3 drops)

Lavender oil (5 drops)

Directions:

1.   Mix ingredients together

2.   Pour into a bottle

3.   Shake thoroughly.

Sweet Honey Soap

Ingredients:

Castile soap (1 lb)

Honey (1/4 lb)

Glycerin (1/4 lb)

Sandalwood essential oil (5drops)

Fine oatmeal (2 tbsp)

Directions:

1.   Grate the soap.

2.   Put some water in the pot

3.   Add the honey, glycerin, the oatmeal and essential oil.

4.   Mix well until soap is dissolved.

5.   Boil for 3 minutes, pour into soap moulds or a deep wet container.

6.   Cut into pieces when it is quite cold.

7.   Leave out until it's dry before storing.

Lavender Soap

Ingredients:

Unscented soap (1)

Dried lavender (1)

Lavender essential oil (3 drops)

Directions:

1.   Grate a bar unscented soap and place inside some water in a bowl.

2.   Place the bowl in a pan of hot water. stir thoroughly until smooth

3.   Add the dried lavender flowers to the soap.

4.   Remove the bowl from pan

5.   Add lavender essential oil

6.   Pour into molds.

Simple Soap Recipe

Ingredients:

Castile Soap Flakes and or/Glycerin Soap (1 lb)

Fennel essential oil (8 drops)

Grapefruit essential oil (14 drops)

Lemon essential oil (8 drops)

Purified Water (1 cup)

Herbal Tea or Hydrosol (1/2 cup)

Directions:

1.   Melt the glycerin in double boiler hydrosol or herbal infusion.

2.   Leave it to cool for a while.

3.   Add essential oil and stir thoroughly.

4.   pour into moulds

5.   Leave to harden and cut into bars.

6.   Use a knife to smooth rough spots.

Herbal Soap

Ingredients:

Block olive or veg. soap (1g)

Loosely chopped herbs (25 g)

Thyme or rosemary essential oil (3 drops)

Finely ground oatmeal (1 tbsp)

Directions:

1.   Grate the soap into a bowl and add the remaining ingredients.

2.   Heat gently till it melts.

3.   Mix well.

4.   Pour soup into each section of an egg box that has been lined with waxed paper.

Basic Lotion Bars

Ingredients:

Beeswax (2 oz)

Almond oil (1 oz)

Cocoa butter (1 oz)

Essential oil (3drops)

Directions:

1.   Melt cocoa butter and beeswax and on the stove in a clean pot.

2.   Once it melts, remove from heat and then add the almond oil.

3.   Mix in the essential oil drop by drop until it's attains the desired scent.

4.   Pour the mixture into a mould.

5.   Leave it to it set fully before using.

3. HAIR CARE RECIPES

Several hair growth care and treatments depend on essential oils. Essential oils are versatile and can work wonders on any type of hair and scalp. Some of them work directly on the hair by helping to strengthen and repair it. Others help to improve the condition of the scalp alone.

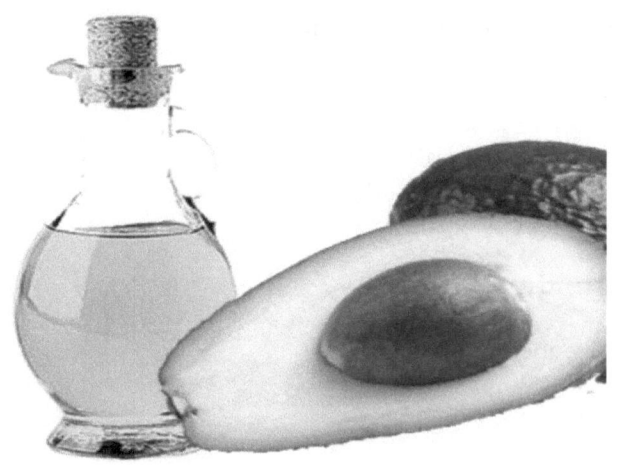

Avocado Hair Moisturizing Recipe

Ingredients:

Half avocado

Peppermint essential oil (few drops)

Oil (1-2 tbsp, optional)

Egg yolk (1-2 tbsp, optional)

Directions:

1.   Mash the avocado up.

2.   Add the essential oil

3.   Shampoo your hair, squeeze the water out and apply mask.

4.   Allow to sit for 15minutes. Rinse off.

5.   Hair will come out super soft and smell real nice.

Homemade Hair Softener/ Growth Recipe

Ingredients:

Thyme essential oil (2 drops)

Cedar essential oil (2 drops)

Rosemary essential oil (3 drops)

Grapeseed (1 ounce)

Jojoba (1 tbsp)

Directions:

1.   Mix all the ingredients in a bowl.

2.   Pour into a tight bottle for easy storage.

3.   Every night, massage the mixture into your scalp.

4.   Rinse in cool water and shampoo the next morning.

5.   For oily hair, 3 times in a week is fine.

6.   This recipe promotes hair growth and softens hair.

Essential Oils For Split Ends

Ingredients:

Sandalwood essential oil (10 drops)

Rosemary essential oil (10 drops)

Directions:

1.   Combine ingredients

2.   Use your fingers to rub them in.

Warm Oil Recipe For Dry Hair

Ingredients:

Aloe Vera gel (2 ounces)

Castor oil (2 ounces)

Rose geranium cedar essential oil (6 drops)

Rosemary essential oil (8 drops)

Ginger essential oil (2 drops)

Directions:

1.   Combine all the ingredients

2.   Warm the mixture and apply to scalp and hair in sections

3.   Use a towel to cover the head and leave it on for an hour.

4.   Wash off.

After Shampooing Rinse: For Dry Hair

Ingredients:

Comfrey oil (2 tsp)

Marshmallow oil (2 tsp)

Parsley essential oil (2 drops)

Sage essential oil (2 drops)

Water (4 cups)

Vinegar (2cups)

Directions:

1.	Combine all the ingredients.

2.	Rinse your hair with this mixture after shampooing.

3.	 Keep it away from your eyes.

4.	 The Rinse can be reused once or twice.

Sweet-Smelling Herbal Shampoo

Ingredients:

Unscented shampoo (2 ounces)

Chamomile essential oil (12 drops)

Lavender essential oil (12 drops)

Directions:

1.	Mix all the ingredients

2.	Shake well before use.

Henna Protein Treatment

Ingredients:

Henna (3 ounces)

Honey (2 tbsp)

Lavender essential oil (24 drops)

Warm water (2 cups)

Olive oil (1 tsp)

Egg (1)

Directions:

1.   Mix all the ingredients

2.   Add this mixture to henna, remove any lumps.

3.   Wet the hair and apply from roots to ends.

4.   Keep the heat in by covering for 1 or 2 hours with a plastic bag and towel.

5.   The henna breaks down and the color becomes darker when you do this but ensure that the henna doesn't dry out.

6.   Rinse several times with warm water, and then apply shampoo and conditioner to it.

7.   Make sure you use gloves and wear an apron to avoid staining your skin.

Deep Endings Essential Oil Treatment

The ends of your hair will be nourished by this revitalizing oil treatment. Its usefulness is more pronounced in the winter when hair tends to rub up against heavy fabrics, including wools.

Ingredients:

Sweet almond, olive or peanut oil (1-3 tsp)

Pure lavender essential oil (2-4 drops)

Note:

The quantity of the peanut, olive or sweet almond oil depends on how long or thick your hair is

Directions:

1.   Combine the oils and apply it to the end of your hair.

2.   Using a clear plastic wrap, wrap the hair and leave for about 30 minutes.

3.   Rinse with Lemon Aid.

Lavender Mist

Ingredients:

Water (½ gallon)

Lavender essential oil (5 drops)

Directions:

1.   Pour the half gallon of water in a large pot.

2.   Cover, boil and let it simmer for 1 hour so as to remove impurities.

(Distilled water can also be used).

3.   Remove from heat and then add the lavender oil

4.   Stir thoroughly, leave to cool

5.   Pour into spritz bottles

Lavender helps to cleanse and revive your hair.

Homemade Hair Conditioner Oil

Ingredients:

Jojoba oil (1 tablespoon)

Rosemary essential oil (3 drops)

Directions:

1.   Mix the essential oil (Rosemary) and jojoba in a small bow

2.   Wet your hair with warm water, apply the mixture and leave it to sit on your hair for 30 minutes.

3.   Wash your hair afterwards.

Scaly Scalp And Dandruff Blend Recipe

Ingredients:

Atlas cedar- wood (2 drops)

Rosemary (2 drops)

Lavender (2 drops)

Tea tree oil (2 drops)

Jojoba (1/2 ounce)

Directions:

1.   Mix all ingredients together.

2.   Apply on scalp

Scented Hair Gel

Ingredients:

Water (1 cup)

Flax seed (2 tbsp)

Essential oil (2 drops)

Directions:

1.   In a small saucepan, mix water and seed.

2.   Bring to boil and then remove from heat.

3.   Allow to set for 30minutes and then strain.

4.   Once cooled, add essential oil

5.   Pour into to a wide-mouthed container with lid.

Quality Hair Treatment

This recipe is ideal for a thicker, smoother and nice-smelling hair.

Ingredients:

Honey (2 spoons)

Olive oil (2 spoons)

Eggs (2)

Rose EO (10 drops)

Lavender EO (5 drops)

Directions:

1.   Combine all ingredients

2.   Apply all over the hair.

3.   leave for an hour

4.   Wash away.

4. LIP BALM RECIPES

Note:

All recipes should be thrown away once it changes odor, texture or color.

Vitamin E Capsule is used as a preservative.

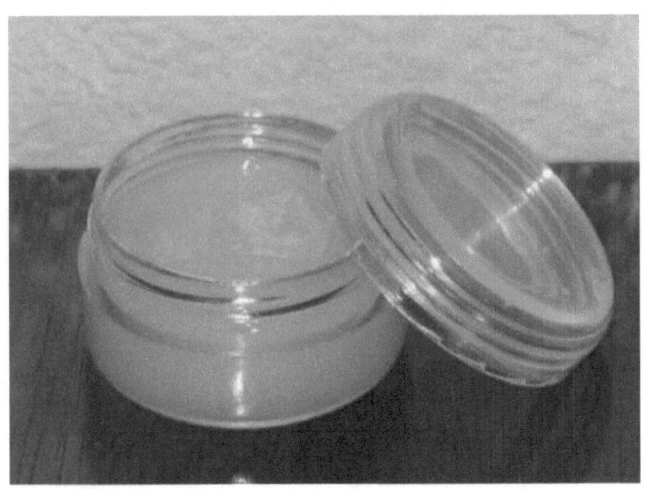

Honey Cocoa Lip Balm

Ingredients:

Olive oil (2 tsp)

Cocoa butter (½ tsp)

Honey (½ tsp)

Beeswax (½ tsp)

Orange essential oil (3 drops)

Vitamin E capsule (1)

Direction:

1.   Place the cocoa butter, oil and beeswax into a glass pan.

2.   Use a hotplate to melt over low heat.

3.   Stir until thoroughly melted. Remove from heat

4.   Add the honey and essential oil into it.

5.   Squeeze the vitamin E capsule into the mixture and stir.

6.   Pour the mixture into fine containers.

Honey Balm

Ingredients:

Almond Oil (3 oz)

Beeswax or Beeswax Pellets (½ oz.)

Honey (2 Teaspoons)

Essential Oil (1-4 Drops)

Vitamin E capsule (1)

Directions:

1.   Mix the beeswax and almond oil together in a bowl.

2.   Place bowl in a pan of water and heat on a stovetop.

3.   Heat until mixture is fully melted, stirring continuously to completely melt the wax.

4.   Remove from heat and add the honey and essential oil in it.

5.   Open the vitamin E capsule, squeeze the contents into it.

6.   Stir the mixture one more time

7.   Allow it to completely cool

8.   Once cool, pour into small plastic containers.

Peppermint Flavored Lip Balm

Ingredients:

Petroleum jelly (2 tbsp)

Beeswax (1 tsp)

Peppermint essential oil (10-14 drops)

Directions:

1.   Melt the petroleum jelly in a small pot.

2.   Add in the beeswax.

3.   Remove from the heat once melted.

4.   Now add the peppermint essential oil.

5.   Pour into a lip pot

6.   Leave to cool.

Tangerine Lip Gloss

Ingredients:

Beeswax (2 tsp)

Honey (1 tsp)

Sweet almond, jojoba or castor oil (7 tsp)

Tangerine essential oil (5 drops)

Directions:

1.   Melt the beeswax and oil until completely melted.

2.   Remove from heat and then add the honey.

3.   Whisk it all up.

4.   When the mixture is almost cool, add the essential oil and mix it up again.

5.   Pour into a container.

Lemon Lip Gloss

Ingredients:

Beeswax (2 tsp)

Honey (1 tsp)

Sweet almond, jojoba or castor oil (7 tsp)

Lemon essential oil (5 drops)

Directions:

1.   Melt the beeswax and oil until completely melted.

2.   Remove from heat and then add the honey.

3.   Whisk it all up.

4.   When the mixture is almost cool, add the essential oil and mix it up again.

5.   Pour into a container.

To make it harder, add more beeswax

Hemp Oil Lip Balm

Ingredients:

Coconut oil (3 tbsp)

Castor oil

Sunflower oil (1 tbsp)

Hemp seed oil (1 tbsp)

Beeswax (1 tbsp)

Honey (1 tbsp)

Peppermint essential oil (few drops)

Directions:

1.   Melt the coconut oil and wax together.

2.   Add the honey and heat for some time.

3.   Stir continuously and add the sunflower and castor oil.

4.   As the mixture thickens, add the peppermint essential oil and the hempseed oil.

5.   Stir until it thickens.

Rosey-Coco Lip Balm Recipe

Ingredients:

Coconut oil (2 Tbsp)

Grated cocoa butter (1 Tbsp)

Dried rosebuds (or any dried flower etc, 1 Tbsp)

Vitamin E oil (1/4 tsp)

Rose, vanilla or lavender essential oil (3 drops)

Directions:

1.   Place the coconut oil in a stainless steel bowl and melt over very low heat.

2.   Once melted, add the roses (or any dried flowers of your choice) and stir thoroughly.

3.   Place on very low heat again for an hour.

4.   Use a cheesecloth or fine-mesh sieve to sieve the oil into a bowl

5.   Clean your original heating bowl and pour the oil back in. Return to heat.

6.   Add the cocoa butter and stir until well melted. Remove from heat.

7.   Add essential oil and vitamin E oil and stir well.

8.   Transfer to a container and leave it for 3 hours to set.

Note:

Remember this is mostly coconut oil so do not put this recipe in a lip balm tube. Do not keep in your pocket, either. Coconut oil liquefies quickly when it is in contact with only a small amount of heat. Even keeping it in a warm place like your body will make it leak all over.

Minty Choc Lip Balm Recipe

Ingredients:

Beeswax pearls or grated beeswax (1 Tbsp)

Coconut oil (1/8 cup)

Shear butter (1/2 Tbsp)

Cocoa butter (1/2 Tbsp)

Honey (1/2 tsp)

Cocoa powder (1 tsp)

Vitamin E oil (1/8 tsp)

Peppermint essential oil (3 drops)

Directions:

1. In a small pot, place the cocoa and Shea butters and add the coconut oil.

2. Heat over extremely low heat for 20 minutes. Stir occasionally. (Do not let the mixture go beyond 175 degrees else the Shea butter will become a little gritty.)

3. Add in the beeswax and stir.

4. When the beeswax is completely melted, remove from heat.

5. Add the honey, cocoa powder, essential oil, and vitamin E, whisking thoroughly the whole time.

6. Once everything is incorporated, transfer to a lip balm tin and leave for 3hours to set.

Sweet Lavender Lip Balm Recipe

Ingredients:

Beeswax pearls or grated beeswax (1 tbsp)

Honey (1 tsp)

Cocoa powder (1 tsp, optional)

Jojoba, olive or almond oil (4 tbsp)

Vitamin E oil (1/4 tsp)

Lavender essential oil (7 drops)

Colored, natural lipstick to give it a hint of color (optional, 1 tsp)

Directions:

1.   Warm the honey, oils and beeswax on very low heat in a small bowl.

2.   Stir until the beeswax is totally melted. Remove from heat.

3.   Quickly whisk in the colored lipstick, cocoa powder, essential oil and vitamin E.

4.   Place the bowl into a pan of ice water and keep on whisking as you add the honey.

5.   Once the honey is fully incorporated, transfer the balm quickly into your lip balm container

6.   Leave to set for 3 hours.

Note

Mineral eye shadow tubs make great lip balm containers so do not throw yours away after use. It's fun to be creative. Match and mix colors until you find the one you love.

Cold Sores Treatment Lip Balm

Ingredients:

 Emu Oil (1 oz)

Almond Oil (1 oz)

Avocado Oil (1 oz)

Beeswax Pellets or Shaved Beeswax (1 /2 oz.)

Aloe Vera Gel (1/4 oz.)

Lavender Essential Oil (6 Drops)

Tea Tree Essential Oil (2 Drops)

Lime Essential Oil (3 Drops)

Directions:

1.   Mix the beeswax, emu, almond and avocado oil together in a bowl.

2.   Heat the bowl in a pan of water on a stove

3.   Stir the mixture repeatedly until the beeswax is melted.

4.   Add the aloe Vera gel.

5.   Remove from heat, add the essential oils and stir.

6.   Stir once more and leave to completely cool.

7.   Transfer into small plastic tins when cool

Sweet Sugar Lip Balm Recipe

Ingredients:

Sweet almond oil (20 ml)

Grated beeswax or beeswax pellets (½ tsp)

Cocoa butter (½ tsp)

Icing sugar (1 tsp)

Vitamin E (1 capsule)

Peppermint, sweet orange or rose essential oil (5 drops)

Directions:

1.   Melt cocoa butter, beeswax and oil in a double boiler

2.   Add the icing sugar and stir so it dissolves.

3.   Remove from heat and then add the vitamin E by puncturing the capsule and pouring oil in.

4.   Add the essential oils, stir again and pour into a lip balm container.

Luscious Lip Balm Recipe

Ingredients:

Filtered, raw beeswax1 tbsp (0.5 oz)

Unscented coconut oil (4 tbsp)

Bergamot essential oil (10 drops)

Directions:

1.   Add beeswax and coconut oil to a glass measuring cup.

2.   Microwave every 30 second until beeswax is melted.

3.   Remove the mixture from the microwave and set aside

4.   Add the essential oil to the mixture, stirring carefully.

5.   Pour slowly into your lip balm tins.

6.   Leave at room temperature to cool and set.

5. HOMEMADE DEODORANTS AND POWDERS

A lot of people react very strongly to store-bought deodorant. Homemade deodorants are a healthy alternative and they cost much less as well.

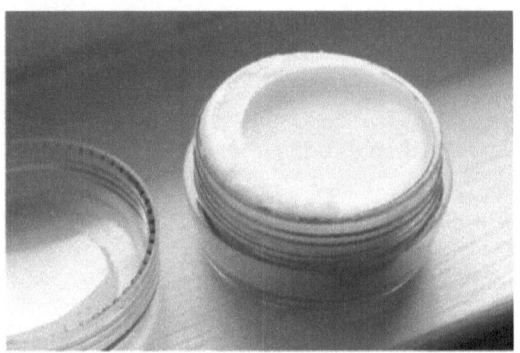

Simple Deodorant Powder

Ingredients:

Coconut Oil (3tbsp)

Baking Soda (3tbsp)

Shea Butter (2tbsp)

Arrowroot (2tbsp)

Essential Oils (5drops)

Directions:

1.   Melt coconut oil and Shea butter in a double boiler over low heat until barely melted

2.   Remove from heat. add arrowroot and baking soda

3.   Mix well

4.   Add essential oils and pour into a glass container for storage

Pineapple Deodorant Powder

Ingredients

Coconut oil (1 tbsp)

Baking soda (1 cup)

Powdered coconut milk (1/2 cups)

Pineapple essential oil (1 tbsp)

Directions

1.   Melt coconut oil and Set aside.

2.   Mix coconut powder and baking soda in a tight-lid container.

3.   Add essential oil and the melted coconut oil.

4.   Use a powder brush or puff to apply the deodorant.

Scented Orange Deodorant Powder

Ingredients:

Baking soda (3 tsps)

Arrowroot powder (2tbs)

Cornflour (2tbs)

Sweet orange essential oil (10 drops)

Neroli essential oil (10 drops)

Directions:

1.	Mix all the dry ingredients in bowl.

2.	Add the essential oils, mix well.

3.	Store in an airtight container.

Fine Thyme Deodorant Powder

Ingredients:

Arrowroot (1 1/2 c)

Baking soda/ bicarbonate of soda (1 cup)

Finely powdered thyme (1/4 c)

Calcium bentonite clay (1/4 c)

Zeolite powder (1 tbsp)

Rosemary essential oil (100 drops)

Thyme essential oil (50 drops)

Directions

1.	Combine all the ingredients except the essential oils in a large bowl.

2.	Blend in a food processor for 20 seconds or whisk by hand.

3.	Slowly add the essential oils to 7 tablespoons of the powder mix. Use a mortar and pestle.

4.	Add oil mixture to the rest of the powder and whirl for 20 seconds in a food processor.

5.	Let the mixture sit for 3 days so that the oils can permeate the powder.

6.   Place in a small jar.

Face Powder Foundation

Ingredients

Cornstarch or arrowroot powder (2 tbsp)

Cinnamon, nutmeg or cocoa powder (1½ tsp, add more as necessary for tinting)

Essential oil (5 drops)

Directions

1.   Mix all the ingredients in a bowl. Stir until well mixed.

2.   Add tint (cocoa powder, cinnamon or nutmeg) until you attain your desired color.

3.   Keep adding any of these tints until you get a similar tone for your skin.

Homemade Probiotic Deodorant

Ingredients:

Cocoa butter (1 tbsp)

Coconut oil (1 tbsp)

Shea butter (1 tbsp)

Beeswax (1 tbsp)

Arrowroot powder (2 1/2 tbsp)

Baking soda (1 tbsp)

Vitamin E oil (1/4 tsp)

Essential oils of choice (15 drops)

Powdered probiotics (2 capsules)

Directions

1.   Melt Shea butter, coconut oil, cocoa butter and beeswax over very low heat.

2.   Remove pot from heat. add baking soda and arrowroot powder into it

3.   Whisk until all powders are dissolved and mixed.

4.   Add essential oils and vitamin E oil. Allow mixture to cool.

5.   Once it is cooled, open the capsules of probiotics and add powder to the mixture.

6.   Stir quickly with spatula to combine.

7.   Add mixture to used but clean deodorant container.

8.   Place in refrigerator to cool and harden.

9.   Store afterwards. Lasts for for3-4 months.

Lemony Deodorant Recipe

Ingredients:

Extra virgin coconut oil (1-1/3 cups)

Beeswax shavings (1-1/2 tablespoons)

Baking soda (1/4 cup)

Arrowroot powder (3/4 cup)

Clay (2 tbsp)

Tea tree essential oil (25 drops)

Lemongrass essential oil (5 drops)

Directions:

1.   Melt beeswax and coconut oil over low heat until barely melted.

2.   Remove from heat and then add the remaining ingredients apart from essential oils.

3.   Leave to cool while stirring continuously until it hardens.

4.   Refrigerate to speed this up. Check and stir frequently.

5.   Add essential oils and thoroughly combine.

6.   Pour into empty deodorant containers.

7.   Leave in a cool location or refrigerate to harden.

8.   For each arm, use about 1/8 teaspoon.

Simply Fresh Deodorant Powder

Ingredients:

Coconut oil (6 tbsp)

Baking soda (4 tbsp)

Arrowroot or cornstarch (4 T)

 Essential oils (5 drops)

Directions:

1.   In a medium sized bowl, mix arrowroot and baking soda together.

2.   Use a fork to mash in coconut oil until well mixed.

3.   add essential oil

4.   Store in a used deodorant container for easy use.

Rich Deodorant Spray

Ingredients:

Vodka (50 ml)

Pure witch hazel (50 ml)

Ylang ylang (10 drops)

Geranium (10 drops)

Bergamot (10 drops)

Sandalwood (10 drops)

Directions:

1.   Add the oils into your glass bottle

2.   Add the vodka and witch hazel.

3.   Close firmly with the sprayer and cap.

4.   Shake thoroughly before each use so as to redistribute the oils.

Homemade Deodorant For Men

Ingredients:

Vodka (50 ml)

Pure witch hazel (50 ml)

Sandalwood (15 drops)

Black pepper (5 drop)

Cypress (10 drops)

Frankincense (5 drops)

Tea tree (5 drops)

Directions:

1.   Add the oils into your glass bottle

2.   Add the vodka and witch hazel.

3.   Close firmly with the sprayer and cap.

4.   Shake thoroughly before each use so as to redistribute the oils.

Herbal Deodorant Powder

Ingredients:

Powdered sandalwood (2 parts)

Powdered white oak bark (1 part)

Powdered lovage root (1 part)

Directions:

1.   Pulverize herbs in a food processor or blender until they are in powdered form.

2.   Transfer powder into an iron skillet. Pan-roast gently.

3.   Pour powdered herbs into a muslin draw-string bags.

4.   Pat bags on your feet or under your arms.

Sage Deodorizing Powder For Foot

Ingredients:

Baking powder (1 tbsp)

Sage essential oil (2 drops)

Directions:

1.   Mix oil and baking powder in a plastic bag.

2.   Shake thoroughly. Set aside to dry.

3.   Break up any formed clumps.

4.   use powder to regularly dust feet

5.   Leave a teaspoon in the shoes overnight.

Fairy Dusting Powder

Ingredients:

Rice Flour (1/2 cup)

Cornstarch (1/2 cup)

Finely ground Rose petals (2 tsp)

Mica, very fine glitter (1/2 tsp)

Essential Oil (3 drops)

Directions:

1.   Mix all the dry ingredients together

2.   Add essential oil and mix thoroughly

3.   Put in an airtight container

6. BODY SCRUB RECIPES

Body scrubs are just great! They work by removing old layers of dead skin, leaving you with a fresh, glowing and healthy skin. There are two major types: salt and sugar. Salt will sting if you have scratches, or rashes. Sugar scrubs are gentler on the skin and also non-stinging so they are ideal for sensitive or irritated skin.

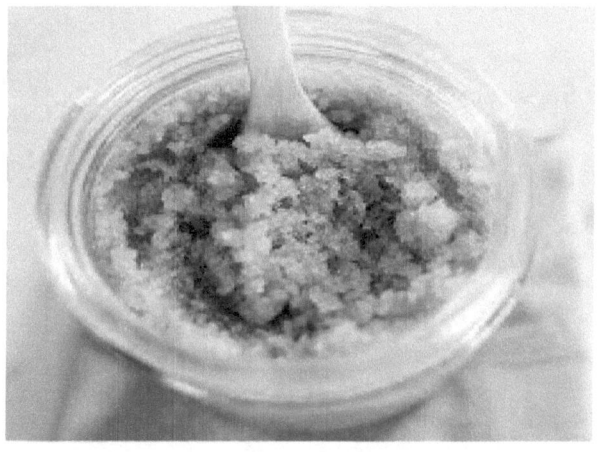

Sweet Sugar Scrub Recipe

Ingredients:

Sugar (3/4 cup)

Honey (1/4 cup)

Vegetable glycerin (1/8 cup)

Olive oil (1/8 cup)

Castile soap (or 1/4 liquid)

Your favorite essential oil (25 drops)

Directions:

1.   Mix all the ingredients together in a bowl

2.   Apply generously after showering, concentrating on areas like the elbows and knees.

3.   Rinse off

4.   Apply any moisturizing body lotion.

Peppermint Sugar Scrub

Ingredients:

White granulated sugar (2 cups)

Almond oil (/4 cup)

Peppermint essential oil (5drops)

Raspberry/pomegranate juice (few drops)

Directions:

1.   Mix the almond oil slowly into the granulated sugar.

2.   Add the peppermint essential oil.

3.   Add drops of pomegranate or raspberry juice.

4.   Mix well until color is even throughout.

Citrus Scrub

Ingredients:

Course Sea salt (1 cup)

Raw sugar (1/2 cup)

Coconut oil (1/2 cup)

Sweet orange essential oil (10 drops)

Grapefruit essential oil (10 drops)

Lemon essential oil (5 drops)

Directions:

1.   Combine the sugar and sea salt in a small jar but don't fill to the top)

2.   Heat the coconut oil on low heat until it liquefies

3.   Remove from heat and add all the essential oils

4.   Pour the essential oil mixture and coconut oil over the sugar and sea salt mixture

5.   Do not stir

6.   apply and massage on the body for some minutes

7.   Rinse

Delectable Scrub

Ingredients:

Organic cane sugar (1 cup)

Celtic sea salt (1/3 cup)

Organic coconut oil (1/2 cup)

Almond oil (2-3 tbsp)

Vitamin E (1 tbsp)

Lavender essential oil (few drops)

Directions:

1.   Combine all ingredients, oils should be last.

2.   Mix well

3.   Apply to body

4.   Massage into skin

5.   Rinse

Banana Sugar Scrub

Ingredients:

Banana (1 ripe)

Granulated sugar (3 tablespoons)

Your favorite essential oil (optional)

Directions:

1.   Use a fork to smash ingredients together in a bowl

2.   Do not over- smash so it won't become too thin

3.   Massage mixture all over your body

4.   Rinse off with warm water.

Peppermint/Lavender Foot Scrub

Ingredients:

Salt (1 cup)

Sweet almond oil (1/3 cup)

Peppermint essential oil (10 drops)

Lavender essential oil (5 drops)

Directions:

1.   Combine ingredients thoroughly in a ceramic or glass bowl.

2.   Apply on feet

3.   Leave for a few minutes

4.   Rinse with warm water

Ginger/ Orange Foot Scrub

Ingredients:

 Brown sugar (1 cup)

Sweet almond oil (1/3 cup)

Orange essential oil (12 drops)

Ginger essential oil (3drops)

Directions:

1.   Combine ingredients thoroughly in a ceramic or glass bowl.

2.   Apply on feet

3.   Leave for a few minutes

4.   Rinse with warm water

Mild Oatmeal Body Scrub

Ingredients:

Finely ground oatmeal (1 cup)

Lavender essential oil (8 drops)

Tangerine essential oil (8 drops)

Rosewood essential oil (8 drops)

Chamomile (4 drops)

Dried lavender petals (1 tbsp, optional)

Directions:

1.   Add oatmeal in a ceramic bowl

2.   Add the essential oils drop by drop. Stir continuously to avoid clumps.

3.   Pour in an airtight jar and refrigerate

4.   Combine one tablespoon of the mixture with some water to form a paste

5.   Gently rub onto skin.

6.   Can be stored for up to a year.

Ginger/ Coconut Oil Sugar Scrub

Ingredients:

Coconut oil (1/4 cup)

Coarsely chopped ginger (1 tbsp)

Carrier oil of choice (1/4 cup)

Granulated sugar (3/4 cup)

Kosher salt (1/4 cup)

Essential oil of choice (1-4 drops)

Directions:

1.   Heat the coconut oil and ginger in a small pan over low heat until liquefied.

2.   Remove from heat. use coffee filter or cheesecloth to press through

3.   Mix warm oils with any carrier oil

4.   Stir in salt and sugar

5.   Add essential oil

6.   Apply to body, massage into skin and rinse

Gentle Magnesium Foot Scrub

Ingredients:

Epsom salt (1 cup)

Olive oil (¼ cup)

Liquid castile soap (1 teaspoon)

Essential oils (10-15 drops)

Directions:

1.   Mix all ingredients in a small bowl.

2.   Add essential oils until desired scent is achieved.

3.   Store in airtight jar

4.   Use a teaspoon sized quantity to exfoliate feet as needed.

5.   Rinse after use.

Cinnamon/ Orange Coffee Scrub Recipe

 Ingredients:

Ground coffee (1 cup)

Salt (1 tbsp)

Ground cinnamon (1 tsp)

Sweet almond oil (1/3 cup)

Grapefruit essential oil (8 drops)

Orange (8 drops)

Peppermint (4 drops)

Directions:

1.   Mix salt, coffee and essential oils in a glass bowl.

2.   Slowly add almond oil slowly and stir continuously until the mixture attains moist sand consistency.

Spicy Sugar Scrub (for Men and Women)

Ingredients:

Organic brown sugar (1 cup)

White granulated sugar (1 cup)

Hazelnut, macadamia nut, almond or soybeans base oil (¾ cup)

Powdered cinnamon (2 tsp)

Powdered ginger (2 tsp)

Powdered nutmeg (2 tsp)

Essential oils (40 drops of any three different types that is good for your skin)

Directions:

1.   Combine all the ingredients except the essential oil in a medium-sized bowl.

2.   Use a whisk to blend all ingredients thoroughly

3.   Add essential oil drop by drop. Blend after each addition.

4.   Spoon mixture into a storage jar with a tight-fitting lid.

5.   Using circular motions, massage ½ cup of scrub onto skin

6.   Rinse.

Exfoliating Sugar Scrub

Ingredients:

White sugar (28g)

Jojoba or Fractionated Coconut Oil (28 mls)

Vegetable Glycerin (5 tsp)

Liquid Castile Soap (28 mls)

Vitamin E Oil (1/2 tsp)

Essential Oil (25 drops)

Directions:

1.   Pour the sugar into a small mixing bowl.

2.   Add the castile soap, oils and glycerin to the sugar.

3.   Mix well.

4.   Add the essential oil and again mix well.

5.   Spoon scrub into a clean tight fitting jar.

Body Buffer

Ingredients:

Jojoba Oil (1/4 cup)

Liquid Soap (1/4 cup)

Very Fine Sea Salt (1/2 cup)

Essential Oil (1/2 tsp)

Directions:

1.   In a small bowl, combine all the ingredients and mix thoroughly.

2.   Pour into a flip-top bottle.

3.   Scrub is in liquid form.

7. BODY LOTIONS, CREAMS & OILS

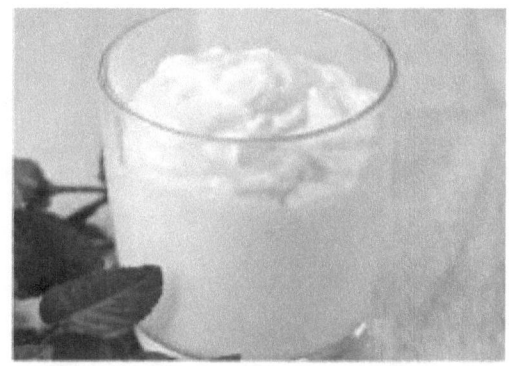

Easy Lotion

Ingredients:

Olive oil (1 cup)

Coconut oil (8 tbsp)

Beeswax, pastilles (8 tbs)

Vitamin E oil (1/2 tsp)

Essential oil (20 drops

Directions:

1.   Combine beeswax pastilles, olive oil and coconut oil in a jar

2.   Put the jar into a saucepan and then fill the saucepan with water, ¾ way up the jar. (be careful, the water mustn't get into the oil mixture)

3.   Heat and stir on the stove over low heat until it melts.

4.   Leave to cool at room temperature or refrigerated.

5.   Add in the essential oil and Vitamin E

6.   While it's cooling, use a fork to stir thoroughly every 15 minutes.

Non-Greasy Homemade Moisturizing Lotion

Ingredients:

Aloe Vera gel (1 cup)

Vitamin E oil (1 tsp)

Grated beeswax (1½ tbsp)

Almond or grape-seed oil (1/2 cup)

Cocoa butter (optional, 1 tbs.)

Essential oils of choice (10 drops)

Directions:

1.   Melt beeswax and oils in a double boiler over low heat.

2.   Combine aloe Vera gel and vitamin E oil in a medium-sized bowl.

3.   Pour the melted oils into a blender. Leave to cool at room temperature.

4.   Once cooled, add the essential oils, put the blender on low speed and slowly pour in the aloe Vera mixture.

5.   Blend the mixture until it looks and feel like lotion.

6.   Pour the lotion into clean jars

7.   Last 6 weeks when refrigerated, less without.

Beeswax Hand Cream

Ingredients:

Beeswax (¼ cup)

Almond oil (¼ cup)

Honey (¼ cup)

Bee pollen (1 tbsp)

Vaseline petroleum jelly (¼ cup)

Glycerin (¼ cup)

Liquid lecithin (2 tbsp)

Lavender essential oil (3 drops)

Directions:

1.   In a double boiler, melt the petroleum jelly and beeswax together.

2.   Add the rest of the ingredients except essential oil and heat for 5 minutes until smooth.

3.   Remove from heat and add the essential oil

4.   While still hot, pour into a jar. It will harden as it cools.

5.   Makes about 1¼ cups.

Coco Beeswax Hand Cream

Ingredients:

Beeswax (¼ cup)

Baby oil (3 tbsp)

Coconut oil (¼ cup)

Rosewood essential oil (3drops)

Glycerin (1/3 cup)

Directions:

1.   In a double boiler, melt the coconut oil and beeswax together.

2.   Add the rest of the ingredients, except essential oil and heat for 5 minutes until smooth.

3.   remove from heat and add the essential oil

4.   While still hot, pour into a jar. It will harden as it cools.

5.   Makes about 1 cup.

Bee Pollen Hand Cream

Ingredients:

Petroleum Jelly (1/2 cup)

Glycerin (1/2 Cup)

Beeswax (1/3 cup)

Bee pollen (2 tablespoons)

Lavender essential oil (3drops)

Directions:

1. In a double boiler, melt the petroleum jelly and beeswax together.

2. Add the glycerin and then heat for a few minutes until the mixture is well heated.

3. Add the bee pollen and essential oil.

4. While still hot, pour into a jar. It will harden as it cools.

5. Makes about 1¼ cups

Beeswax Cold Cream

Ingredients:

Beeswax (1/3 cup)

Glycerin (¼ cup)

Liquid lecithin (1 tbsp)

Baby oil (¼ cup)

Almond oil (¼ cup)

Bee pollen (1 tbsp)

Essential oil of choice (3drops)

Directions:

1. Melt beeswax over a double boiler.

2. Add the rest of the ingredients, except essential oil and heat until smooth.

3. add the essential oil

4.   While still hot, pour into a container. It will harden as it cools.

5.   Makes about 1½ cups

Beeswax Almond Hand Cream

Ingredients:

Beeswax (¼ cup)

Almond oil (½ cup)

Coconut oil (½ cup)

Rosewater (¼ cup)

Essential oil of choice (3drops)

Directions:

1.   Melt the coconut oil and beeswax over a double boiler. Add the remaining ingredients

2.   Add the rest of the ingredients, except essential oil and heat until smooth.

3.   add the essential oil

4.   While still hot, pour into a container. It will harden as it cools.

5.   Makes about 1½ cups

Stretch Mark Oil

Ingredients:

Rose (4 drops)

Rosemary (1 drop)

Camellia Oil (1/2 teaspoon)

Sesame Oil (1/2 teaspoon)

Vitamin E Oil (1/2 teaspoon)

Wheat Germ Oil (1/2 teaspoon)

Directions:

Massage on stretch mark areas.

Lush Body Oil

Ingredients:

Sunflower Oil (4 oz)

Hazelnut Nut Oil (1 tsp)

Evening of Primrose Oil (1 tsp)

Macadamia Nut Oil (1 tsp)

Vitamin E Oil--20 drops

Directions:

1.   Mix all ingredients together

2.   Store in tightly covered bottle.

3.   Refrigerate for longer shelf life.

Anti-Wrinkle Oil

Ingredients:

Rose (2 drops)

Rosemary (1 drop)

Rosewood (2 drop)

Sandalwood (3 drops)

Directions:

1.   Mix together and apply as needed.

Spot Beater Oil

Ingredients:

Castor Oil (1 oz)

Emu Oil (0.5 oz)

Tea Tree EO (30 drops)

Directions:

1.   Mix together and then package.

2.   Oil easily soaks into skin

Moisturizing Anti-Aging Face Cream

Ingredients:

Beeswax (4 tsp)

Olive oil (4 tbsp)

Shea butter, coconut oil or mango butter (2tbsp)

Water or green tea (8 tbsp)

Jojoba (1 tbsp)

Glycerin (1 tbsp)

Essential oil (10 to 15 drops)

Directions:

1.   Melt the beeswax and oil in a double boiler. Stir until well mixed.

2.   Add the shear butter, stir until it well melted into the wax.

3.   Remove from the heat and then whip with a hand-held mixer while adding the aloe Vera, green tea and glycerin.

4.   Continue whipping until the cream becomes light and fluffy. Leave it to cool to room temperature.

5.   Blend in the essential oil, stir until fully combined.

6.   Pour into a container and seal.

7.   This recipe makes about 227g of anti-aging face cream.

Note:

Since this recipe contains no preservative, keep unused cream refrigerated for about 6 months. Alternatively, keep in a cool place for about 3 months.

Remove cream from container, using washable or cosmetic spatulas and not your fingers to prevent contamination.

Foot Lotion For Aching Feet

Ingredients:

Almond oil (1 tbsp)

Olive oil (1 tbsp)

Wheat germ oil (1 tbsp)

Eucalyptus essential oil (12 drops)

Directions:

1.   Combine all ingredients in a bottle.

2.   Shake thoroughly.

3.   Just rub into the heels and feet.

4.   Store in a cool dry place.

Dry Hand Lotion

Ingredients:

Unscented Lotion (8 oz)

Patchouli (20 drops)

Sandalwood (40 drops)

Borage (20 drops)

Carrot Tissue (5 drops)

Directions:

1.   Pour the lotion into a bowl.

2.   Add the oils and mix thoroughly.

3.   Put the lotion back into the bottle.

Heavy Duty Hand Cream

Ingredients:

Shaved beeswax (2 Tbsp)

Carnuba wax (1/2 tsp)

Jojoba oil 2 (tbsp)

Aloe Vera gel (1 tsp)

Vitamin E oil (10 drops) or Vitamin E capsules (4)

Any essential oil (1 drop)

Directions:

1.   Melt the beeswax, carnuba wax, Jojoba oil and Aloe Vera in a pot either on the stove or in the microwave.

2.   Remove from heat, beat until cool and add Vitamin E oil before the mixture thickens.

3.   Continue beating until mixture becomes creamy.

4.   Add essential oil and keep beating until cream has totally cooled.

5.   Spoon cream into a jar and store in a cool dark place

Lemon Facial Cleansing Cream

Ingredients:

Beeswax (1 tbsp)

Jojoba oil or Coconut oil (3 tbsp)

Witch hazel (1 tbsp)

Lemon juice (1 tbsp)

Bicarbonate of soda 1/8 tsp. (basically a pinch)

Lemon essential oil (6 drops)

Directions:

1.   In a saucepan, melt the beeswax over low heat.

2.   Add the coconut oil (or jojoba) and beat for 5 minutes with a hand mixer.

3.   Heat the witch hazel and lemon juice in another saucepan until warm.

4.   Add in the bicarbonate of soda to dissolve.

5.   Add this liquid mixture to the cream, beat until well combined.

6.   Leave the cream to cool for a while

7.   Add the lemon essential oil.

8.   Spoon into a container.

8. PERFUMES RECIPES

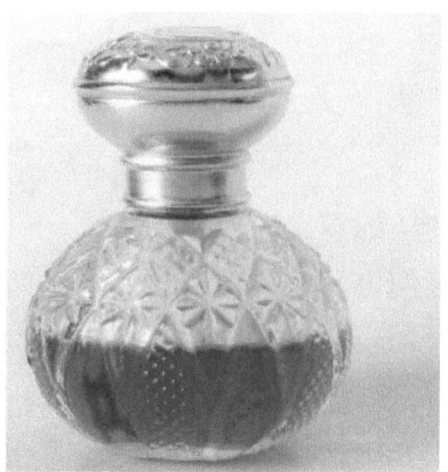

Oriental Nights Perfume

Ingredients:

Sandalwood (4 drops)

Musk (4 drops)

Frankincense (3 drops)

Jojoba oil (2 teaspoons)

Directions:

1. Combine all the ingredients together.

2. Shake well.

3. allow to settle for 12 hours

4. Store in a cool dry area.

Whispering Drops Perfume

Ingredients:

Distilled water (2 cups)

Vodka 3 (tbsp)

Sandalwood essential oil (5 drops)

Bergamot essential oil (10 drops)

Cassis essential oil (10 drops)

Directions:

1. Combine all the ingredients together.

2. Shake well.

3. allow to settle for 12 hours

4. Store in a cool dry area.

Citrus Bloom Body Splash

Ingredients:

Distilled water (2 cups)

Vodka (3 tbsp)

Finely chopped orange and lemon peel (1tablespoon each)

Lemon verbena essential oil (5 drops)

Mandarin essential oil (10 drops)

Orange essential oil (10 drops)

Directions:

1.   Add the fruit peels with the vodka in a jar.

2.   Cover and leave for a week.

3.   Strain the liquid and then add the water and essential oils to the liquid.

4.   Leave for 2 weeks but shake the jar once a day.

5.   Keep in a cool dark area.

Relaxing Summer Body Spray

Ingredients:

Witch hazel (1 tbsp)

Lemon Extract (1 tbsp)

Cucumber Extract (1 tbsp)

Water (1 cup)

Directions:

1.   Combine all ingredients

2.   Transfer to a pump spray bottle

Soothing Body Perfume

Ingredients:

Sandalwood (25 drops Base note)

Rose, Jasmine or Neroli (3 drops of Middle note)

Jojoba (2 tbsp)

Directions:

1.   Blend all the oils together.

2.   Store in an airtight dark-colored glass jar

3.   Leave for some days to mature.

4.   Dab only a drop onto your pulse points.

5.   Use sparingly due to the heavy concentration of essential oils.

www.ingramcontent.com/pod-product-compliance
Lightning Source LLC
Chambersburg PA
CBHW050504290526
45786CB00006B/2425